Slow Cooker for Beginners

The Slow Cooker Recipe Book
with Quick and Healthy Recipes
incl. Vegan and Vegetarian (UK Version)

[1st Edition]

Adam Bailey

Table of contents

Slow Cooker for Beginners

Introduction

The slow cooker has been around for decades, making the busy lifestyle of millions a little easier. These simple devices are built simple and are easy to use. The unit itself is built to heat from underneath, and, with a tight-fitting lid, you are ensured to keep the heat locked in. This makes for an environment that is perfect for cooking meats. Built with an earthenware insert and a tight-fitting lid, the mighty slow cooker does so much more than most people know.

Over the generations, slow cookers have fallen out of the limelight, but don't worry, they always make a comeback. They are a handy tool to have in your kitchen arsenal, and they are a part of the everyday life of millions across the globe.

Tips and Tricks for How to Use a Slow Cooker

Still, when using this simple device there are tips and techniques that you can use to make this kitchen staple even more efficient.

- Not All Meat is Created Equally

  As its name implies, the slow cooker cooks over a longer period of time than other cookers. This means that delicate cuts can get obliterated, so it is better to choose a tougher cut of meat. It is also great for larger cuts of meat like roasts or whole chickens. The way that this unit is built, there is no way you will overcook or dry out your meal if you are using the right cut of meat.

- Brown Before You Cook

  Adding an extra step like browning can have two benefits to your slow cooker meal. The first is that it will look better on the plate, but the bigger benefit is the enhancement of the overall flavor. Searing your meat creates all-new flavor profiles. Plus, you can deglaze the pan and get a whole wealth of deeper flavors that will make the meal just a bit better.

- Too Much of Anything is Bad

  Every slow cooker will come with a set of guidelines about how much is optimal to put in it. Most models stick with the two-thirds idea. This means you should only fill your slow cooker until it is two-thirds full. If you overcrowd or fill the slow cooker, it will be harder for the unit to reach its temperature, and that could mean longer cooking times and could also be a food safety problem. Many people also add too many liquids. The process that happens in the unit will produce juices, and, since there is little to no evaporation, you will be fine adding fewer liquids than you think you need.

- Defrost Ingredients First

  You can cook small things like peas while they are still frozen, but, when it comes to the meaty part of the meal, making sure that it is thoroughly defrosted is a good idea. This is more about food safety as opposed to what the unit can do.

- Dairy is Last in the Pool

  Dairy, when placed in the cooker and cooked too long, will begin to break down and separate. Thus, it is much better to add cheese, cream, and such dairy products toward the end of the cooking process so that you steer clear of unwanted pools of cheese, grease, or milk solids.

- Remember to Always Be Safe

  Though this kitchen appliance can be left on all day or even overnight, you should still think about safety. For instance, if there was a power outage and the pot of meat stood out all day, it may be best to just throw it out and start fresh.

- Some other fun tips…

  - Use a non-stick cooking spray to coat the inside of the slow cooker. This will make cleaning up afterward a lot easier.

- You can also invest in liner bags specifically made for slow cookers that will also make clean up faster.
- The high setting for most slow cookers is about 280 F (138 C), while the low setting tends to hover around 170 F (77 C).
- Typically, the ratio of cooking is one hour on high equals two hours on low.
- Try adding any fresh herbs at the end of the cooking process to help liven up the flavors.
- Any heartier vegetables, like potatoes, should go on the bottom of the slow cooker so they will cook faster and more evenly.

These are just a few of the many tips and tricks you can learn in regards to the slow cooker.

How to Clean a Slow Cooker

Making sure you clean and maintain your slow cooker properly will extend the life of this versatile kitchen appliance. The first and most vital thing is to make sure that the unit is off and has cooled down before you start cleaning it. The lid and insert can be cleaned in the traditional way with hot water and soap, or they can be placed in the dishwasher. However, if you choose to clean it the old-fashioned way, there are a few tips that will help you:

- Stay away from harsh abrasive cleaners and cleaning tools. You should use the basic scrubbing brush, and, if you have bits that are hard to get off, try using a plastic spatula.
- Try using vinegar or gentle cleaners to remove dirt and gunk.
- You have to use hot water to clean your insert. Cold water, just like with any other dish, will just not do the trick.
- Never take the base that does the heating and immerse it in water. It is electric, and this will mess up the unit and make it dangerous to use. Instead, once it has cooled down, wipe it with a damp rag and then dry thoroughly.

Other than keeping it clean, you will want to make sure all the parts are in tip-top shape. So, if something starts to act a little funky, don't just replace the unit. Look to see if you can find replacement parts, as this will save you time and money.

RECIPES FOR BREAKFAST

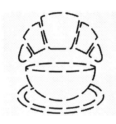

Breakfast Casserole

Serves: 6-8

Nutritional Facts: Calories: 588 | Carbs: 14.6g | Protein: 32.7g | Fat: 45.8g

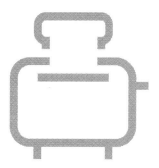

Ingredients:

- 1 bag of frozen hash brown potatoes (32 oz./907g)
- 1 lb. bacon (454g)
- 1 sm. onion, diced
- 8 oz. shredded cheddar cheese (227g)
- ½ bell pepper, red, diced
- ½ bell pepper, green, diced
- 12 eggs
- 1 cup of milk (237ml)

Directions:

1. Cut up bacon and cook. Drain the grease and set bacon aside. Dice vegetables.

2. Layer half of the ingredients (except eggs and milk) into the slow cooker and then repeat layers for the remainder of the ingredients.

3. Crack the eggs into a medium bowl and add milk. Whisk until combined and frothy.

4. Pour mixture over ingredients in slow cooker and season with salt and pepper.

5. Cook for 4 hours on low or 8 hours on warm. Once done cooking, the dish is ready to serve.

Egg, Spinach, and Ham Casserole

Serves: 6-8

Nutritional Facts: Calories: 150 | Carbs: 3.2g | Protein: 8.7 | Fat: 11.4g

Ingredients:

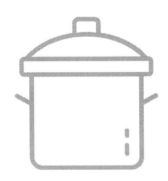

- 6 large eggs
- ½ tsp. salt
- ¼ tsp. pepper
- ½ cup of Greek yogurt (118ml)
- ½ tsp. thyme
- ½ tsp. onion powder
- ½ tsp. garlic powder

- ⅓ cup of mushrooms, diced (50g)
- 1 cup of baby spinach (237g)
- 1 cup of pepper jack cheese, shredded (237g)
- 1 cup of ham, diced (237g)

Preparation:

1. Crack eggs into a medium bowl and add in all the ingredients except themushrooms, spinach, cheese, and ham. Whisk until thoroughly combined.
2. Now, add in the remaining ingredients.
3. Spray the slow cooker with non-stick cooking spray and pour the mixture into the slow cooker.
4. Cook on high for up to 2 hours or until the eggs have set.
5. Cut and serve.

Overnight Cinnamon Apple Oatmeal

Serves: 8

Nutritional Facts: Calories: 179 | Carbs: 18.8g | Protein: 3.2g | Fat: 13.3g

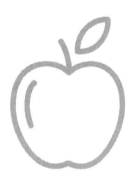

Ingredients:

- ♦ 1 cup of oats, steel-cut (237ml)
- ♦ 1 ½ cups of coconut milk (355ml)
- ♦ 1 ½ cups of water (355ml)
- ♦ 2 apples, peeled and diced
- ♦ 2 tbsp. brown sugar
- ♦ 1 tsp. cinnamon
- ♦ ¼ tsp. sea salt

Directions:

1. Spray the inside of the slow cooker with a non-stick cooking spray.
2. Place all ingredients into the slow cooker and stir until combined.
3. Cook on low for up to 7 hours or until oats are to your liking.
4. Serve with toppings (cinnamon/brown sugar, nuts, or fresh fruit) of your choice.

Breakfast Quinoa

Serves: 4

Nutritional Facts: Calories: 220 | Carbs: 36.9g | Protein: 7.9g | Fat: 4.6g

Ingredients:

- ♦ 1 cup of quinoa, uncooked (237ml)
- ♦ 2 cups of water (474ml)
- ♦ 1 cup of coconut milk, canned (237ml)
- ♦ 2 tbsp. maple syrup/raw honey
- ♦ ¼ tsp. salt

Preparation:

1. Rinse the quinoa in a fine mesh colander under cold water for a minute.

2. Add in all the ingredients into the slow cooker and cover. Cook on low for about 8 hours.

3. Serve with your choice of toppings (nuts, fruit, honey, etc.) and/or a splash of milk.

Breakfast Tater Tot Casserole

Serves: 8

Nutritional Facts: Calories: 414 | Carbs: 29g | Protein: 21g | Fat: 23g

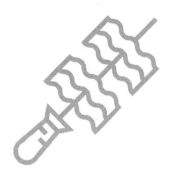

Ingredients:

- 1 bag of frozen tater tots (32oz./907g)
- 1 lb. turkey sausage, ground (454g)
- 6 large eggs
- 2 tbsp. heavy cream
- ½ tsp. thyme, dried
- ½ tsp. garlic powder
- ¼ tsp. salt
- ⅛ tsp. pepper
- 1 cup of Colby Jack cheese, shredded (237g)

Directions:

1. Spray inside of slow cooker with no-stick cooking spray. Then, add ⅔ bag of tater tots.

2. In a medium bowl, combine eggs with the remaining ingredients (except the sausage and cheese) and whisk until combined. Then pour into the slow cooker.

3. Heat a skillet over medium-high heat and brown the sausage. Make sure to break it into small pieces. Then add to the slow cooker.

4. Pour remaining tater tots into the slow cooker and cover with cheese.

5. Cook covered on high for 2-3 hours or low for 4-6 hours. Then serve.

Hash Brown Casserole

Serves: 6-8

Nutritional Facts: Calories: 169 | Carbs: 20.1g | Protein: 4.2g | Fat: 8.4g

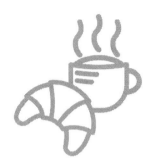

Ingredients:

- 3 tbsp. butter
- ¼ cup of mushrooms, chopped (38g)
- ¼ cup of onion, chopped (38g)
- ¼ tsp. garlic powder
- 3 tbsp. flour
- 1 cup of milk
- ½ cup of sour cream
- 1 bag of shredded hash browns, frozen (20oz./567g)
- 1 cup of cheddar cheese, shredded (83g)
- 1 tsp. salt
- ¼ tsp. pepper

Preparation:

1. Heat a small saucepan over medium heat and melt the butter. Then, add mushrooms and onions into the pan. Sauté until tender. Next, add garlic powder and flour into the pan. Whisk until thick paste forms. Cook for 1 minute.

2. Slowly add milk while whisking. Reduce heat and let simmer until thickened. Remove from heat and add sour cream.

3. Pour sauce into the slow cooker and top with hash browns and cheese. Add salt and pepper and combine ingredients together well.

4. Cover and cook for up to 3 hours. Then, remove the lid and cook for half an hour.

5. Turn off and serve with your choice of toppings.

Cheesy Potatoes

Serves: 8

Nutritional Facts: Calories: 367 | Carbs: 32.7g | Protein: 21.5g | Fat: 16.4g

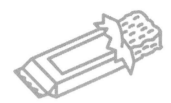

Ingredients:

- ♦ 3 large potatoes, peeled and diced
- ♦ 1 bell pepper, red, diced
- ♦ 1 bell pepper, green, diced
- ♦ 1 onion, diced
- ♦ 1 package ofandouille sausage, thinly sliced
- ♦ 1 ½ cups of cheddar cheese, shredded (125g)
- ♦ ½ cup of sour cream (118ml)
- ♦ ¼ tsp. oregano, dried
- ♦ ¼ tsp. basil, dried
- ♦ 1 can of cream of chicken soup
- ♦ Salt and pepper to taste
- ♦ 2 tbsp. parsley, fresh, chopped

Directions:

1. Combine all the ingredients (except the parsley) into the slow cooker. Then, stir in cream of chicken soup and season to taste.

2. Cook covered on low heat for 4-5 hours or high heat for 2-3 hours.

3. Then, serve garnished with parsley

French Toast w/ Nutella and Caramelized Bananas

Serves: 8

Nutritional Facts: Calories: 137 | Carbs: 14.4g | Protein: 4.7g | Fat: 6.4g

Ingredients:

- 1 loaf of challah bread, cubed
- 6 large eggs
- 2 cups of almond milk (474g)
- 1 tsp. cinnamon, ground
- 1 tbsp. vanilla extract
- 2 tbsp. Nutella
- Pinch of salt
- 1 tbsp. butter, unsalted
- 4 bananas, sliced
- 1 tbsp. brown sugar

Preparation:

1. Cube the bread and place in the slow cooker.

2. Combine the eggs, milk, cinnamon, vanilla extract, Nutella, and salt into a medium mixing bowl and whisk until thoroughly combined. Pour over cubed bread and mix until bread is soaked with the mixture.

3. Cook covered for 2 hours on high. Make sure to check every hour and stir the mix for even cooking.

4. Slice your bananas and place them in a bowl with brown sugar. Mix until bananas are coated.

5. In a sauté pan over medium-high heat, melt some butter and add in the bananas. Cook for two minutes on each side or until brown on both sides.

6. Scoop out French toast and top with bananas and more Nutella and then serve.

Slow Cooker Caramel Rolls

Serves: 8

Nutritional Facts: Calories: 103 | Carbs: 10.1g | Protein: .5g | Fat: 7g

Ingredients:

♦ 1 package of cinnamon rolls, refrigerated

♦ 4 tbsp. butter

♦ ½ cup of brown sugar (97g)

Directions:

1. Spray the inside of the slow cooker with non-stick cooking spray.

2. Heat a small saucepan over medium heat and melt the butter with the brown sugar. Cook this until the sauce is thick and smooth.

3. Now, place packaged rolls in the bottom of the slow cooker and pour the sauce over the top.

4. Cook covered on high for about 1 ½ hours.

Monkey Bread

Serves: 10

Nutritional Facts: Calories: 86 | Carbs: 7.8g | Protein: .4g | Fat: 6.2g

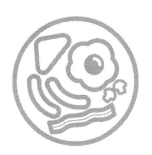

Ingredients:

♦ 2 cans of refrigerated cinnamon rolls

♦ ¼ cup of granulated sugar (50g)

♦ 1 tsp. cinnamon

♦ ½ cup of brown sugar (97g)

♦ ½ cup of unsalted butter, melted (97g)

Directions:

1. Open can of cinnamon rolls and cut each roll into six pieces. Combine granulated sugar and cinnamon in a large freezer bag and toss the pieces of dough into it. Seal the bag and shake to coat the dough.

2. In a small saucepan, melt the butter and brown sugar over a medium heat. Then, spray the inside of the slow cooker with non-stick cooking spray.

3. Take half of the sugar/cinnamon-coated dough and place them on the bottom of the slow cooker. Pour half of the melted butter / brown sugar mixture over the top.

4. Next, add the rest of the dough pieces and the other half of the melted butter mixture and cover.

5. Cook on high for about two hours or until the edges start to brown. Turn off the cooker and let cool for five minutes and then serve.

MAIN DISH WITH MEAT

Asian Broccoli & Beef

Serves: 4-6

Nutritional Facts: Calories: 470 | Carbs: 40.4g | Protein: 40.8g | Fat: 16.3g

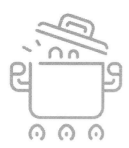

Ingredients:

- 1 ½ lb. sirloin steak, sliced thin (680g)
- 1 cup of beef broth, low sodium (237ml)
- ½ cup of soy sauce, low sodium (118ml)
- ½ cup of brown sugar (97g)
- 2 tbsp. sesame oil
- 1 tbsp. sriracha
- 3 cloves garlic, minced
- 3 green onions, sliced thin
- 2 tbsp. cornstarch
- 2 cups of broccoli florets (303g)
- Sesame seeds
- Jasmine rice, cooked

Directions:

1. Combine steak, broth, soy sauce, brown sugar, sesame oil, sriracha, garlic, and green onions in a slow cooker. Cook covered on low for about 3 ½ hours or until beef is tender.

2. Spoon some of the broth into a small mixing bowl and add in the cornstarch. Whisk until combined and pour into the slow cooker. Stir well, and then add in broccoli. Cook covered for another 20 minutes.

3. Serve with rice and garnish with sesame seeds and green onions.

Beef Tacos

Serves: 8

Nutritional Facts: Calories: 178 | Carbs: 5.9g | Protein: 23.3g | Fat: 7.5g

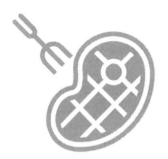

Ingredients:

- 1 small beef chuck roast
- 1 large onion, diced
- 4 cloves garlic, chopped
- 3 limes, juiced
- 1 tbsp. chili powder
- 1 tbsp. cumin, ground
- 1 tbsp. oregano, dried
- 4 cups of chicken broth, low sodium (946ml)
- 20 small corn tortillas
- Sour cream, green onions, red onions, and lime wedges for serving

Directions:

1. Add all the ingredients except the tortillas and toppings into a slow cooker and pour the broth over mixture. Cover and cook on low for 8 hours.

2. Remove roast and onions, then shred roast and onions, placing the shredded beef in a large bowl. Spoon broth over the meat until the beef is moistened but not wet.

3. Heat corn tortillas over flame and top with beef. Serve with toppings and garnishes.

Beef-Stuffed Peppers

Serves: 4

Nutritional Facts: Calories: 644 | Carbs: 33g | Protein: 51.5g | Fat: 34.1g

Ingredients:

- 1 lb. ground beef (454g)
- 1 can of black beans, drained and rinsed
- 1 can of diced fire-roasted tomatoes, drained
- 2 cups of Monterey Jack cheese, shredded (167g)
- 1 cup of white rice, cooked (178g)
- 1 cup of frozen corn, defrosted (171g)
- 1 tsp. cumin
- 1 tsp. chili powder
- ½ tsp. garlic powder
- ½ tsp. oregano
- Salt & pepper to taste
- 4 bell peppers, tops, and seeds removed
- 1 tbsp. cilantro, chopped
- Sour cream

Directions:

1. Cook rice and beef per the desired method. Then, combine beef, tomatoes, 1 cup of cheese, rice, corn, cumin, chili powder, and oregano together in a large mixing bowl. Mix until combined well and season with salt and pepper for taste.

2. Trim the peppers and remove seeds. Then, stuff each one with the mixture and place in slow cooker stuffing side up. Cover and cook on high for 3 hours.

3. Top with remaining cheese and cook for another 10 minutes or until the cheese melts.

4. Remove from slow cooker, top with sour cream, garnish with cilantro, and serve.

Beef Bourguignon

Serves: 6

Nutritional Facts: Calories: 619 | Carbs: 7g | Protein: 81.6g | Fat: 28.7g

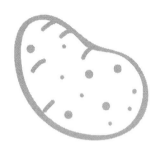

Ingredients:

- ♦ 1 medium beef chuck roast, cut into chunks
- ♦ 3 tbsp. olive oil, extra virgin
- ♦ 1 cup of red wine (237ml)
- ♦ 1 cup of beef broth (237ml)
- ♦ 2 cups of mushrooms, sliced (341g)
- ♦ 2 large carrots, slice into disks
- ♦ 1 large onion, diced
- ♦ 2 cloves garlic, chopped
- ♦ 3 sprigs thyme, fresh
- ♦ 3 sprigs rosemary, fresh
- ♦ 1 bunch asparagus, trimmed and quartered
- ♦ Parsley, fresh, chopped

Directions:

1. Heat the oil in a large skillet over medium-high heat and then add beef (may have to do in batches). Sear the beef for about 3 minutes per side. In between batches, use red wine to deglaze and scrape up any bits with a wooden spoon. Pour that mixture into the slow cooker along with the completed beef. Repeat until all beef is seared.

2. Then, add the broth, vegetables, remaining red wine, and herbs. Cover and cook on high for about 7 hours or until beef is so tender it is easy to shred.

3. About half an hour before the beef is done, remove herbs and add in asparagus. Then cook until asparagus is tender.

4. Serve garnished with parsley.

Pot Roast w/ Potatoes

Serves: 4

Nutritional Facts: Calories: 469 | Carbs: 46.5g | Protein: 45g | Fat: 13.4g

Ingredients:

- 1 ½ lb. beef chuck (680g)
- Salt and pepper for taste
- Olive oil, extra virgin (for drizzling)
- 1 tbsp. tomato paste
- 2 tbsp. vinegar, apple cider
- 2 cups of beef broth, low sodium (474ml)
- 1 onion, chopped (1")
- 1 can of cannellini beans
- 1 lb. baby potatoes (454g)
- 10 cloves garlic
- 1 bay leaf
- ½ cup parsley, fresh, chopped (42g)

Directions:

1. Heat a large skillet over high heat. Pat beef dry and season generously with salt and pepper. Add oil to hot skillet and sear beef until golden brown on both sides. Then, move to the slow cooker.

2. Combine tomato paste, vinegar, salt, and pepper in a small mixing bowl. Whisk until thoroughly combined. Then, pour into the slow cooker. Add in the rest of the ingredients except the parsley. Cook on low for about 8 hours or until the meat is tender.

3. Remove the bay leaf and serve garnished with parsley.

Chicken Cacciatore

Serves: 6

Nutritional Facts: Calories: 880 | Carbs: 36.4g | Protein: 32g | Fat: 70.3g

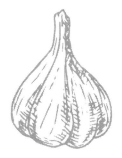

Ingredients:

- ◆ 2 lbs. chicken thighs, bone-in, skin-on (907g)
- ◆ Salt and pepper for taste
- ◆ 2 bell peppers, chopped
- ◆ 8 oz. mushrooms, sliced (57g)
- ◆ 2 cloves garlic, minced
- ◆ 1 can of crushed tomatoes
- ◆ ½ cup of chicken broth (118ml)
- ◆ 1 tsp. oregano, dried
- ◆ ¼ tsp. pepper flakes
- ◆ ⅓ cup of capers (48g)
- ◆ 8 oz. linguini (227g)

Directions:

1. Salt and pepper both sides of the chicken thighs and place them in the slow cooker. Add in the rest of the ingredients except the capers and pasta. Cook, covered, on low for 6-8 hours or high for 3-4 hours, or until chicken is cooked through.

2. Remove chicken and add capers into the sauce. Stir until mixed. Then, serve chicken on a bed of pasta with sauce spooned over the top.

Creamy Parmesan Chicken

Serves: 6

Nutritional Facts: Calories: 825 | Carbs: 18.7g | Protein: 20g | Fat: 75g

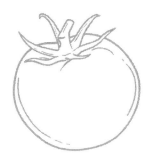

Ingredients:

- 2 lbs. chicken thighs, bone-in, skin-on (907g)
- Salt and pepper for taste
- 1lb. baby potatoes, halved (454g)
- 1 bell pepper, red, sliced
- ½ cup of chicken broth, low sodium (118ml)
- ½ cup of heavy cream (118ml)
- ½ cup of Parmesan, grated (142g)
- 2 tbsp. butter, melted
- 1 tsp. oregano, dried
- 1 tsp. garlic powder
- Basil, fresh, sliced thin

Directions:

1. Heat a large skillet with 1 tbsp. butter in it over medium-high heat. Season both sides of the chicken generously and then add to skillet. Sear on both sides until golden brown.

2. While you are doing that, combine the rest of the ingredients into the slow cooker. Once the chicken is done, place the chicken on top of themixture.

3. Cook on high for 3-4 hours or until potatoes are tender and chicken is cooked thoroughly.

4. Serve garnished with parsley and Parmesan.

Rotisserie Chicken

Serves: 4-6

Nutritional Facts: Calories: 285 | Carbs: 4.9g | Protein: 48.7g | Fat: 6.7g

Ingredients:

- ♦ Cooking spray
- ♦ 2 tbsp. brown sugar, packed
- ♦ 1 ½ tsp. chili powder
- ♦ 1 tsp. paprika, smoked
- ♦ 1 tsp. thyme, fresh
- ♦ 1 whole chicken
- ♦ Salt and pepper for taste

Directions:

1. Spray the inside of the slow cooker. Ball up several pieces of aluminum foil to create a rack.

2. Combine brown sugar, chili powder, paprika, and thyme in a small mixing bowl and whisk together. Then, pat the chicken dry and season with salt and pepper. After that, rub the entire chicken down with the brown sugar mixture.

3. Place chicken facing breast down in the slow cooker and cook on high for 2 ½ to 3 ½ hours or until juices run clear.

4. Remove from slow cooker and place on a baking sheet. Broil in oven for 4 minutes for crispy skin. Next, let sit for 10 minutes and then serve.

Apple Cider Braised Pork

Serves: 8

Nutritional Facts: Calories: 388 | Carbs: 13.5g | Protein: 23.6g | Fat: 25.9g

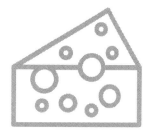

Ingredients:

- ♦ 1 pork shoulder roast, boneless
- ♦ Salt and pepper for taste
- ♦ 1 tbsp. vegetable oil
- ♦ 2 shallots, sliced
- ♦ 1 stalk of celery, chopped
- ♦ ½ cup of vinegar, apple cider (118ml)
- ♦ 2 ½ cups of apple cider (592ml)
- ♦ 4 cloves garlic, peeled
- ♦ 1 bay leaf
- ♦ 1 ½ tsp. Dijon mustard
- ♦ 1 pinch of cayenne pepper
- ♦ 2 tbsp butter, cold, cubed
- ♦ 1 tbsp. fresh herbs of choice

Directions:

1. Season pork roast with salt and pepper generously. Then, in a large skillet, heat oil over high heat and searpork on all sides. Move pork to the slow cooker.

2. Reduce the heat under the skillet and add the shallots and celery. Cook until they begin to soften and then pour in the apple cider vinegar. Cook, scraping up the bits until the liquid is nearly gone.

3. Pour shallots over pork in the slow cooker and add the apple cider, garlic, and bay leaf. Then, cover and cook on low for about 6 hours or untilpork is tender. Turn pork over and cook for another 2 hours.

4. Remove pork and set on aluminum foil. Take the liquid from slow cooker and strain through a fine-mesh strainer into a saucepan. Bring sauce to a boil and then decrease heat. Skim the fat and let it reduce until it is only a quarter of what was originally in the pan.

5. Then, remove the sauce and add in the mustard and cayenne pepper. Slowly add in cold butter, whisking until completely combined. Sprinkle in your fresh herbs, salt, and pepper for taste.

6. Next, cut the roast into ¼" thick pieces and serve with sauce spooned over top.

Bacon Ranch Turkey

Serves: 8

Nutritional Facts: Calories: 194 | Carbs: 3g | Protein: 8.2g | Fat: 15.4g

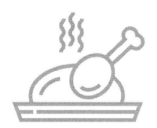

Ingredients:

♦ Cooking spray

♦ ¼ cup of butter, softened

♦ 1 package of ranch dressing mix

♦ 1 turkey breast, bone-in, rinsed and patted dry

♦ 6 slices of bacon, thick-cut

♦ 1 cup of beer, light-colored (237ml)

Directions:

1. Spray inside of slow cooker with non-stick cooking spray.

2. Add butter and half of the ranch mix to a small bowl and mix until thoroughly combined. Loosen the skin on the turkey breast and spread butter mixture under the skin. Move the turkey to the slow cooker, placing it skin side up.

3. Sprinkle the rest of the ranch packet over the turkey breast. Place bacon slices evenly across turkey breast and pour beer around the breast.

4. Cook on high for 1 hour. Then, reduce the temp and cook for another 8 hours or until the turkey is tender. Take it out, let it rest, then slice and serve.

MAIN DISH WITH SEAFOOD & FISH

Shrimp Scampi

Serves: 4

Nutritional Facts: Calories: 168 | Carbs: 2g | Protein: 19g | Fat: 9g

Ingredients:

- ¼ cup of chicken broth (59ml)
- ¼ cup of lemon juice, fresh (59ml)
- ½ cup of white wine (118ml)
- 2 tbsp. olive oil
- 2 tsp. garlic, chopped
- 2 tsp. parsley, minced
- 1 lb. shrimp, raw, large, thawed (454g)

Directions:

1. Combine chicken broth, wine, lemon juice, oil, garlic, and parsley in the slow cooker. Then, add in the shrimp.

2. Cover and cook on low for 2 ½ hours. Then, remove shrimp and serve with some of the juice and crusty bread or pasta.

Cheesy Grits w/ Shrimp

Serves: 4

Nutritional Facts: Calories: 440 | Carbs: 18g | Protein: 33.4g | Fat: 26g

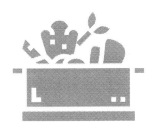

Ingredients:

- 2 cups of grits (319g)
- Salt and pepper for taste
- ¼ cup of heavy cream (59ml)
- 1 cup of cheese, shredded (83g)
- 2 tbsp. butter, unsalted
- 2 tsp. hot sauce
- 1 lb. shrimp, peeled, cooked, deveined (454g)
- 1 tbsp. chives, chopped
- 8 cups of water (1.9L)

Directions:

1. Combine grits with water and 1 ½ tsp. of salt in the slow cooker and whisk together. Cover and cook on low for 6 hours or until liquid is gone.

2. Then, add in cream, cheese, butter, and hot sauce. Stir until cheese is completely melted.

3. Salt and pepper for taste and place the shrimp on top and cook covered for about another 5 minutes or until shrimp is warmed through.

4. Serve with a garnish of chives.

Fish Curry

Serves: 4-6

Nutritional Facts: Calories: 403 | Carbs: 11.2g | Protein: 20.2g | Fat: 33g

Ingredients:

♦ 3 oz. canola oil (80ml)

♦ 1 onion, chopped fine

♦ 2 cloves garlic, minced

♦ 2 small green chilies, seeded and minced

♦ 1" ginger, fresh, peeled and grated (2.5cm)

♦ 1 tbsp. cumin, ground

♦ 2 tsp. coriander, ground

♦ 2 tsp. mustard seeds

♦ 2 tsp. turmeric, ground

♦ 2 tomatoes, chopped and seeded

♦ 1 tbsp. sugar

♦ Salt for taste

♦ 2 lbs. fish fillets, mild, firm, white, cut into chunks (1kg)

♦ 3 tbsp. cilantro, fresh, chopped

♦ 1 ½ cups of water (375ml)

Directions:

1. Place slow cooker insert on the stovetop over medium-high heat. Add oil and heat until hot. Add in onion and cook until golden. Then, add in garlic, chilies, ginger, cumin, coriander, mustard, and turmeric and cook until it becomes fragrant.

2. Then, add in the tomatoes, sugar, and 1 tsp. of salt. Cook until tomatoes begin to release juices. Pour in 1 ½ cups of water to deglaze the pan. Allow to come to a boil.

3. Next, place slow cooker insert back into the slow cooker and let cook on low for two hours. Remove the lid and gently stir in fish chunks. Replace lid and let cook for another 30 minutes or until the fish is opaque. Season with salt and serve over jasmine rice garnished with cilantro.

Maple Salmon

Serves: 6

Nutritional Facts: Calories: 426 | Carbs: 14.7g | Protein: 40.1g | Fat: 22g

Ingredients:

- 6 Salmon fillets
- ½ cup of maple syrup (118ml)
- ⅛ cup of lime juice, fresh (31ml)
- ¼ cup of soy sauce (59ml)
- 2 tsp. crushed garlic
- 1 tsp. ginger, minced

Directions:

1. Place fillets in the slow cooker.

2. Combine remaining ingredients in a small mixing bowl and whisk until combined. Pour over salmon.

3. Cover and cook on high for 1-2 hours, depending on whether the fish is thawed or not. Then, remove from slow cooker and serve with rice or steamed vegetables.

Halibut w/ Lemon & Dill

Serves: 2

Nutritional Facts: Calories: 683 | Carbs: 131g | Protein: 26g | Fat: 9g

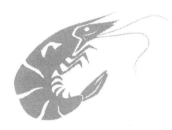

Ingredients:

- ♦ 12 oz. halibut (340g)
- ♦ Salt and pepper for taste
- ♦ 1 tbsp. lemon juice, fresh
- ♦ 1 tbsp. olive oil
- ♦ 1 tbsp. dill fresh

Directions:

1. Pull out an 18" (46cm) sheet of aluminum foil and spray it with non-stick cooking spray. Place halibut fillet in the middle of the foil and salt and pepper the fish on all sides.

2. Add the lemon juice, oil, and dill into a small mixing bowl and whisk until combined. Pour the mixture over the top of the halibut.

3. Bring up the edges of the foil and create a packet around the fish. Place packet in the slow cooker and cook on high for 1 ½ to 2 hours.

4. Open packet and make sure the fish is flakey. Then, serve.

VEGAN AND VEGETARIAN

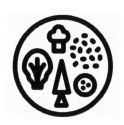

Pinto Bean Enchiladas

Serves: 4 - 6

Nutritional Facts: Calories: 467 | Carbs: 69g | Protein: 14g | Fat: 17g

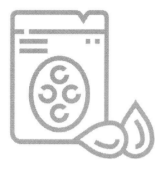

Ingredients:

Enchilada sauce:

- ♦ 3 tbsp. olive oil
- ♦ 2 tbsp. flour, all-purpose
- ♦ 3 tbsp. chili powder
- ♦ 1 ½ tsp. cumin, ground
- ♦ 1 tsp. garlic powder
- ♦ 2 cups of water (473ml)
- ♦ 2 tbsp. tomato paste

Enchiladas:

- ♦ 1 can of pinto beans, rinsed and drained
- ♦ 1 cupof corn, fresh (171g)
- ♦ 1 medium onion, diced
- ♦ 3 cloves garlic, minced
- ♦ 2 tbsp. green chilies, canned
- ♦ 2 tsp. cumin, ground
- ♦ 1 tsp. oregano, dried
- ♦ Salt for taste
- ♦ 6 medium tortillas, flour

Directions:

1. Start by making the sauce. Heat a saucepan over medium heat with oil in it. Then, slowly whisk the flour in. Once it begins to bubble, add in the chili powder, cumin, and garlic powder and whisk them into the flour mixture. After that, add in the water and tomato paste. Turn up the heat and bring sauce to a boil. Then, lower the heat and let sauce simmer for 10 minutes. Stir occasionally until it thickens. Remove from heat and allow to cool down.

2. Next, prepare the filling. Combine the beans, corn, onion, garlic, chilies, cumin, and oregano together in a medium mixing bowl. Season with salt and stir to combine.

3. Spoon about half of the sauce into the bottom of the slow cooker. Then, place the tortilla on a workspace and fill with filling. Roll the tortilla tightly and place seam down into the slow cooker. Repeat for all the tortillas. Next, pour the remaining sauce over the enchiladas.

4. Cook on high for 2 to 3 hours. Then, remove and serve with your choice of avocado slices, cilantro, sour cream, or scallions.

Vegetable Pot Pie

Serves: 6

Nutritional Facts: Calories: 489 | Carbs: 59g | Protein: 12g | Fat: 24g

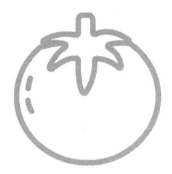

Ingredients:

♦ 7 cups of chopped veggies of your choice (1250g)

♦ ½ cup of onions, diced (85g)

♦ 4 cloves garlic, diced

♦ 5-6 sprigs of thyme, fresh, leaves removed

♦ ¼ cup of flour (31g)

♦ 2 cups of chicken broth (473ml)

♦ ¼ cup of cornstarch (31g)

♦ ¼ cup of heavy cream (59ml)

♦ Salt and pepper for taste

♦ 1 frozen puff pastry sheet, thawed

♦ 2 tbsp. butter

Directions:

1. Clean and cut up the vegetables. Add them and the onion and garlic to the slow cooker. Toss with flour until coated. Slowly stir in broth until combined thoroughly. Cover and cook on high for 3-4 hours.

2. Combine cornstarch and ¼ cup (59ml) of water and whisk until smooth. Then, stir that mixture into the vegetables in the slow cooker. Add in cream, as well, and replace the lid. Continue cooking until the mixture thickens.

3. Preheat oven to 400 F (204 C). Remove from slow cooker and place in a 9 x 13 (22 x 33) baking dish and cover with puff pastry. Melt butter in a small saucepan and brush over the top of the pastry.

4. Bake for 10 minutes or until pastry is golden and puffy.

Eggplant Parmesan

Serves: 12

Nutritional Facts: Calories: 258 | Carbs: 23g | Protein: 16g | Fat: 12g

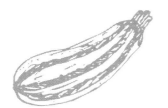

Ingredients:

- 4 lbs. eggplant (1.8kg)
- 1 tbsp. salt
- 3 large eggs
- ¼ cup of milk (59ml)
- 1 ½ cup of breadcrumbs (160g)
- 3 oz. Parmesan cheese, grated (85g)
- 2 tsp. Italian seasoning
- 4 cups of marinara sauce, jarred (946ml)
- 16 oz. mozzarella, sliced (454g)
- Basil, fresh, chopped

Directions:

1. Peel eggplant and slice into ⅓" (.84cm) rounds. Lay out on a baking sheet lined with a paper towel. Salt both sides and allow to sit for 30 minutes. Then, pat dry.

2. Ladle ½ cup (118ml) marinara sauce on the bottom of the slow cooker.

3. In a medium mixing bowl, add the eggs and milk. Whisk until combined. Then, in a separate bowl combine breadcrumbs, Parmesan cheese, and Italian seasoning. Dip eggplant in the egg mixture and then in the bread crumbs. Layer these slices in the slow cooker. Then, top with 1 cup (118ml) of sauce and mozzarella cheese. Repeat the process two more times.

4. Cook on low for 8 hours. When done, serve garnished with basil.

Vegan Jambalaya

Serves: 6 - 8

Nutritional Facts: Calories: 383 | Carbs: 69.6g | Protein: 13.8g | Fat: 6.2g

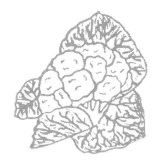

Ingredients:

- 1 tbsp. olive oil
- 1 green bell pepper, diced
- 2 celery sticks, diced
- 1 medium onion, diced
- 3 cloves garlic, minced
- 1 ½ cups of tomatoes, diced (225g)
- 4 – 5 cups of vegetable broth (946ml – 1182ml)
- 2 tbsp. paprika
- 2 tbsp. cumin, ground
- 2 tsp. oregano, dried
- 2 tsp. pepper
- 2 tbsp. hot sauce
- 2 cups of brown rice, long-grained (273g)
- 1 can of kidney beans
- 2 cups of vegan sausage, chopped (364g)
- 2 – 3 scallions, chopped

Directions:

1. Combine all the ingredients except the rice, beans, scallions, and sausage into the slow cooker. Cook covered on low for 4 or 5 hours. Stir occasionally.

2. After that, add in the rice and turn the heat to high. Stir and then replace the lid and continue cooking until rice is tender and liquid is absorbed.

3. Next, add in beans and sausage and cook for another two minutes or until the beans and sausage are heated thoroughly. Make sure to stir into the rice mixture.

4. Serve garnished with scallions.

Vegetable Curry w/ Chickpeas (Vegan)

Serves: 4

Nutritional Facts: Calories: 292 | Carbs: 55.2g | Protein: 13.1g | Fat: 4.7g

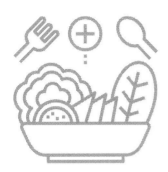

Ingredients:

- 4 cups of cauliflower, florets (728g)
- 2 cups of Brussel sprouts, quartered (303g)
- 1 sweet potato, peeled and diced
- 1 red bell pepper, diced
- 1medium onion, diced
- 1 can of chickpeas, drained and rinsed
- 1 can of tomato sauce, low sodium
- ½ cup of coconut milk (118ml)
- ½ cup of vegetable broth (118ml)
- 1 tbsp. cumin, ground
- 1 tbsp. curry powder
- 1 tbsp. turmeric, ground
- ½ tsp. cayenne
- ½ cup of peas, frozen (85g)
- Salt and pepper to taste

Directions:

1. Combine all the ingredients except the peas in the slow cooker and cook on low heat for 8 hours. Just before serving, stir in peas and let cook until heated through.

2. Serve over rice and garnish with cilantro, scallions, and/or sriracha.

VEGTABLES

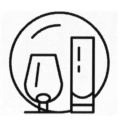

Spiced Autumn Acorn Squash

Serves: 4

Nutritional Facts: Calories: 235 | Carbs: 31g | Protein: 7g | Fat: 9g

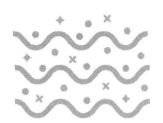

Ingredients:

- ¾ cup of brown sugar, packed (146g)
- 1 tsp. cinnamon, ground
- 1 tsp. nutmeg, ground
- 2 small acorn squash, halved and seeded
- ¾ cup of raisins (128g)
- 4 tbsp. butter
- ½ cup of water (118ml)

Directions:

1. Combine in a small mixing bowl the sugar, cinnamon, and nutmeg and mix well. Then, spoon mixture on top of squash halves. Sprinkle with raisins and top each with a tablespoon of butter. Tightly wrap each in aluminum foil.

2. Pour water into the slow cooker and place squash in it. Make sure to place them cut side up. Cook on high, covered, for 3 ½ to 4 hours or until squash is tender. Add thyme in the slow cooker. Then, pour in ¼ cup (59ml) of Marsala wine. Cover and cook on low until vegetables are tender (about 4 hours).

Baked Potatoes

Serves: 6

Nutritional Facts: Calories: 217 | Carbs: 38g | Protein: 5g | Fat: 6g

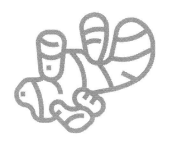

Ingredients:

♦ 6 medium potatoes, russet

♦ 3 tbsp. butter softened

♦ 3 cloves garlic, minced

♦ 1 cup of water (237ml)

♦ Salt and pepper for taste

Directions:

1. Wash potatoes and pierce with fork multiple times. In a small mixing bowl, mix the butter and garlic together. Rub the potatoes with the mixture. Wrap each tightly with aluminum foil. Pour water into the slow cooker and add potatoes into the slow cooker. Cover and cook on low for 8 hours or until tender.

2. Remove from slow cooker and serve with toppings of your preference.

Chickpea Tagine

Serves: 12

Nutritional Facts: Calories: 127 | Carbs: 23g | Protein: 4g | Fat: 3g

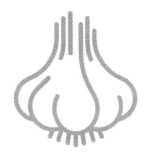

Ingredients:

- 1 small butternut squash, peeled and cut into cubes
- 2 medium zucchini, cut into ½ inch (1.3cm) pieces
- 1 medium red bell pepper, chopped
- 1 medium onion, chopped
- 1 can of chickpeas, rinsed and drained
- 12 apricots, dried, halved
- 2 tbsp. olive oil
- 2 cloves garlic, minced
- 2 tsp. paprika
- 1 tsp. ginger, ground
- 1 tsp. cumin, ground
- ½ tsp. salt
- ¼ tsp. cinnamon, ground
- 1 can of crushed tomatoes
- 2 – 3 tsp. harissa
- 2 tsp. honey
- ¼ cup of mint leaves, fresh, chopped (27g)

Directions:

1. Combine the first six ingredients in the slow cooker.

2. Heat oil in a medium skillet over medium heat. Add in the garlic, paprika, ginger, cumin, salt, pepper, and cinnamon. Cook until the spices become fragrant. Add tomatoes, harissa, and honey. Bring to boil. Pour tomato mixture over vegetables in the slow cooker and stir until combined. Cover and cook on low until vegetables are tender and the sauce has thickened (about 5 hours). Stir in mint.

3. Serve garnished with mint, olive oil, and honey.

Spaghetti Squash Italian-Style

Serves: 4

Nutritional Facts: Calories: 195 | Carbs: 31g | Protein: 9g | Fat: 6g

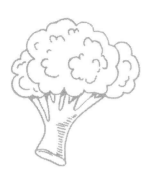

Ingredients:

♦ 1 cup of mushrooms, sliced (150g)

♦ ½ tsp. salt

♦ ½ tsp. oregano, dried

♦ ¼ tsp. pepper

♦ ¾ cup of mozzarella cheese, shredded (63g)

Directions:

1. Cut squash in half lengthwise. Remove seeds and fill with mushrooms and tomatoes. Sprinkle seasonings over the top. Place in the slow cooker.

2. Cover and cook on low until squash is tender (about 6 – 8 hours). Sprinkle with cheese. Replace lid and cook until cheese is melted, and then serve.

SOUP, STEWS, & CHILIS

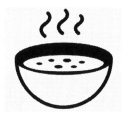

Potato Bacon Soup

Serves: 10

Nutritional Facts: Calories: 309 | Carbs: 33g | Protein: 11g | Fat: 16g

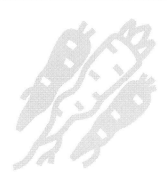

Ingredients:

- 5 lbs. potatoes, peeled and chopped (2.3kg)
- ½ lb. bacon, cooked and crumbled (227g)
- 1 onion, chopped
- 1 cup of sour cream (215g)
- 3 cans of chicken broth
- 10 ¾ oz. cream of chicken soup (305g)

Directions:

1. Place all ingredients into the slow cooker and stir together.
2. Cover and cook on low for 8-10 hours.

Chicken Tortilla Soup

Serves: 8 - 10

Nutritional Facts: Calories: 45 | Carbs: 9g | Protein: 2.2g | Fat: 1.3g

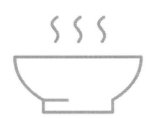

Ingredients:

- ♦ 4 chicken breasts, skinless, boneless
- ♦ 2 cans of diced tomatoes & chilies w/ lime juice & cilantro
- ♦ 1 small can of green chilies, chopped
- ♦ 1 can of black beans, drained and rinsed
- ♦ 1 can of tomato sauce
- ♦ 1 cup of salsa (215g)

Directions:

1. Place the chicken in the slow cooker.
2. Combine all the rest of the ingredients in the slow cooker. Cover and cook on low for 8 hours.
3. Remove chicken when cooked and shred the chicken. Next, replace the chicken back into the slow cooker for another 30 minutes.
4. Serve in bowls with a garnish of your choice.

Broccoli Cheddar Soup

Serves: 6 - 8

Nutritional Facts: Calories: 707 | Carbs: 56.6g | Protein: 65.5g | Fat: 32g

Ingredients:

- ♦ 3 tbsp. butter
- ♦ 1 small onion, diced
- ♦ 4 - 5 cloves garlic, minced
- ♦ 2 bags broccoli, frozen
- ♦ 1 cup of carrots, diced (171g)
- ♦ 32 oz. chicken broth (907g)
- ♦ 1 cup of water (237ml)
- ♦ ½ tsp. pepper
- ♦ 1 tsp. salt
- ♦ 1 can of evaporated milk
- ♦ 8 oz. cream cheese, cubed (227g)
- ♦ 4 cups of cheddar cheese, shredded (333g)

Directions:

1. Heat a skillet on medium-high heat with oil. Melt butter and then sau-té onion and garlic until softened. Then, add this mixture to the slow cooker.

2. Next, add in broccoli, carrots, broth, water, salt, and pepper. Cook on low for 6 hours. After that, add in the milk, cream cheese, and cheddar cheese. Stir, replace the lid, and cook for another half an hour.

3. Next, take soup from the slow cooker in batches and process through the blender. Add soup back to slow cooker and serve.

Brunswick Stew

Serves: 8 - 10

Nutritional Facts: Calories: 579 | Carbs: 55g | Protein: 48g | Fat: 19g

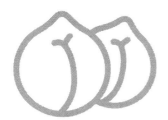

Ingredients:

- 2 cups of lima beans (129g)
- 2 cups of corn (341g)
- 1 lb. okra, sliced (454g)
- 2 cups of potatoes, diced (364g)
- 1 onion, diced
- 2 cans of diced tomatoes
- 2 cups of chicken, cooked, shredded (280g)
- 2 cups of pork, cooked, shredded (280g)
- 1 tbsp. seasoned salt
- 1 cup of chicken stock (237ml)
- 1 cup of BBQ sauce (237ml)

Directions:

1. Add all the ingredients into the slow cooker.
2. Cover and cook on high for 4 hours or until vegetables are tender. Stir and then serve over cornbread.

Beef Stew

Serves: 8

Nutritional Facts: Calories: 277 | Carbs: 31g | Protein: 29g | Fat: 5g

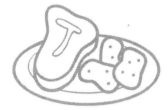

Ingredients:

- 2 lbs. beef stew meat, cubed (907g)
- 2 potatoes, peeled, cubed
- 3 stalks celery, chopped
- 4 carrots, peeled, chopped
- 2 onions, quartered
- 2 cups of tomato juice (473ml)
- ⅓ cup of barley (34g)
- 1 tbsp. sugar
- 1 tbsp. salt
- ½ tsp. basil, dried
- ¼ tsp. pepper

Directions:

1. Combine all the ingredients in the slow cooker. Cover and cook on low for 8 hours or until vegetables are tender and the meat is cooked.

Slow Cooker Chili

Serves: 8 -10

Nutritional Facts: Calories: 357 | Carbs: 12.9g | Protein: 42.2g | Fat: 15.8g

Ingredients:

- 1 lb. ground beef, browned and drained (454g)
- 1 lb. beef stew meat, cubed (454g)
- 1 onion, chopped
- 1 green bell pepper, chopped
- 1 can of kidney beans, drained and rinsed
- 1 can of diced tomatoes with juice
- 1 can of diced tomatoes with green chilies and juice
- 1 can of tomato paste
- 3 tsp. chili powder
- 2 tsp. cumin
- 1 packet of ranch dressing mix
- 3 cloves garlic, peeled and smashed
- 1 can of beef broth

Directions:

1. Combine all ingredients in a slow cooker and stir well.
2. Cover and cook on low for 8 hours. Then, serve garnished with cheese, sour cream, and/or scallions.

Chicken Chili

Serves: 8 - 10

Nutritional Facts: Calories: 164 | Carbs: 9g | Protein: 25.4g | Fat: 10.4g

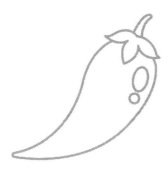

Ingredients:

- ♦ 3 large chicken breasts
- ♦ Salt, pepper, & garlic powder
- ♦ 3 tbsp. olive oil
- ♦ 1 onion, diced
- ♦ 1 jalapeno, diced
- ♦ 1 packet of ranch dressing mix
- ♦ 1 packet of taco seasoning
- ♦ 1 can of pinto beans
- ♦ 1 can of great northern beans
- ♦ 1 can of diced green chilies

Directions:

1. Heat the oil in a large skillet over medium-high heat. Season, cut up chicken with salt, pepper, and garlic powder. Add chicken, onions, and jalapeno into skillet and sauté until lightly browned.

2. Add chicken mixture into the slow cooker with the rest of the ingredients. Stir until mixed and cook on low for 8 hours.

3. Then, serve topped with cheese and/or cilantro.

DESSERT & SNACKS

Peanut Butter Chocolate Cake

Serves: 10

Nutritional Facts: Calories: 607 | Carbs: 57g | Protein: 13g | Fat: 39g

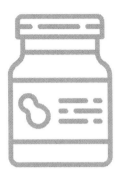

Ingredients:

- 1 devil food cake mix
- 1 cup of water (237ml)
- ½ cup of butter, unsalted, melted (118ml)
- 3 eggs
- 1 package of peanut butter cups
- 1 cup of creamy peanut butter (230g)
- 3 tbsp. powdered sugar
- 10 bite-size peanut butter cups

Directions:

1. In a large mixing bowl, combine the cake mix, water, butter, and eggs until smooth. Stir in the mini peanut butter cups. Spray the inside of the slow cooker with non-stick cooking spray and then add the batter evenly.

2. Cover and cook on high for 2 hours. Then, remove insert from heat.

3. In a small saucepan, combine the peanut butter cups. Cook until melted and smooth. Then, add powdered sugar and whisk until smooth.

4. Pour over warm cake and top with peanut butter cups. Serve and enjoy.

Apple Pear Crisp

Serves: 8

Nutritional Facts: Calories: 319 | Carbs: 51.2g | Protein: 4.1g | Fat: 13.4g

Ingredients:

- 4 apples, peeled and cut into ½" (1.3cm) slices
- 3 pears, peeled and cut into ½" (1.3cm) slices
- ⅓ cup of brown sugar, light
- 1 tbsp. flour, all-purpose
- 1 tbsp. lemon juice, fresh
- ½ tsp. cinnamon, ground
- ¼ tsp. salt
- Pinch of ground nutmeg

Topping

- ¾ cup of flour, all-purpose
- ¾ cup of old fashioned oats
- ½ cup of pecans, chopped
- ⅓ cup of brown sugar, light
- ½ tsp. cinnamon, ground
- ½ tsp. salt
- 8 tbsp. butter, unsalted, cubed

Directions:

1. Make the topping by combining all the ingredients except the butter into a medium mixing bowl. Mix well and then add the butter in. Toss to coat and then use your fingers to begin to work the ingredients together until it is a coarse crumble.

2. Spray the inside of the slow cooker with non-stick cooking spray. Then, place apples and pears into the slow cooker. Add in the brown sugar, lemon juice, flour, cinnamon, salt, and nutmeg and stir until combined. Then, gently sprinkle topping over the top and press softly into the batter.

3. Drape a clean towel over the slow cooker and cook on low heat for 2-3 hours. Then, remove the dish towel and cook another hour or until the topping has browned and apples are soft. Serve warm.

Cheesecake

Serves: 20

Nutritional Facts: Calories: 278 | Carbs: 20g | Protein: 4g | Fat: 20g

Ingredients:

Crust

- ♦ 1 ½ cups of graham cracker crumbs (341g)
- ♦ 6 tbsp. butter, melted

Filling

- ♦ 24 oz. cream cheese (680g)
- ♦ 1 ½ cups of sour cream (323g)
- ♦ 1 ¼ cups of granulated sugar (251g)
- ♦ 5 large eggs
- ♦ 3 tbsp. flour, all-purpose
- ♦ 1 tbsp. vanilla extract
- ♦ ½ tsp. salt

Directions:

1. Line a slow cooker with parchment paper and spray with non-stick cooking spray. Turn slow cooker on low. In a food processor, pulse graham crackers into a fine crumb. Then, pour melted butter into pulse to combine. Pour crumbs into the bottom of the slow cooker and press down making an even layer.

2. After cleaning out the food processor, combine cream cheese and sugar and pulse until a smooth consistency. Scrape the bowl and add in the sour cream, eggs, flour, vanilla, and salt. Blend until thoroughly combined and smooth.

3. Pour the filling over the crust. Cover and cook for 5-7 hours on low or until a toothpick is inserted and comes out clean. Make sure to wipe moisture off lid frequently.

4. Then, remove the insert and place it in the refrigerator. Let cool for about three hours. Next, using the parchment paper, lift the cheese-cake out carefully. Peel the paper, slice, and serve.

Snack Mix

Serves: 12

Nutritional Facts: Calories: 81 | Carbs: 43g | Protein: 10g | Fat: 15g

Ingredients:

- 9 cups of Chex cereal (545g)
- 2 cups of pretzels (303g)
- 1 cup of Cheerios (61g)
- 1 cup of peanuts (152g)
- 6 tbsp. butter, melted and hot
- 1 tbsp. seasoned salt
- ¼ cup of Worcestershire sauce (59ml)
- 1 tsp. garlic powder

Directions:

1. Add all the cereal and nuts into the slow cooker.

2. Then, in a small mixing bowl, combine melted butter, seasoned salt, and garlic powder. Mix until combined and salt has dissolved. Then, stir in the Worcestershire sauce.

3. Drizzle sauce over cereal mix and toss until coated evenly. Cook on low for 3 hours, stirring every hour. Then, remove the mix from slow cooker and lay out on a baking sheet until cool. Serve fresh or store in a sealed container for snacking later.

Jalapeno Popper Taquitos

Serves: 8

Nutritional Facts: Calories: 678 | Carbs: 50g | Protein: 42g | Fat: 33g

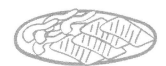

Ingredients:

- 4 chicken breasts, boneless, skinless
- 8 oz. cream cheese (227g)
- ⅓ cup of jalapenos, jarred, sliced (36g)
- 1 tsp. garlic powder
- 1 tsp. salt
- 1 tsp. cumin
- 16 small tortillas
- 1 ½ cups of cheese, shredded (125g)

Directions:

1. Combine chicken, ½ cup (118ml) of water, cream cheese, jalapenos, garlic powder, salt, and cumin to the slow cooker. Cover and cook on low for 6-8 hours.

2. Preheat oven to 425 F (218 C) and spray a baking sheet with non-stick cooking spray. Then, remove the chicken and shred it. Place back in slow cooker mixture and stir until combined well.

3. Heat tortillas in the microwave for a few seconds to make them pliable. Then, sprinkle cheese in the middle of each tortilla. Place a few tablespoons of the mixture over the cheese and roll tightly.

4. Place the taquitos on the baking sheet and bake for up to 15 minutes or until cheese is melted.

5. Serve warm with toppings and sauce of choice.

KETO RECIPES

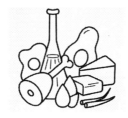

Balsamic Chicken

Serves: 10

Nutritional Facts: Calories: 238 | Carbs: 7g | Protein: 25g | Fat: 12g

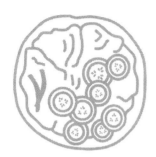

Ingredients:

- 4 - 6 chicken breasts, boneless, skinless
- 2 cans of diced tomatoes
- 1 medium onion, sliced thin
- 4 cloves garlic
- ½ cup of balsamic vinegar (118ml)
- 1 tbsp. olive oil
- 1 tsp. oregano, dried
- 1 tsp. basil, dried
- 1 tsp. rosemary, dried
- ½ tsp. thyme, dried
- Salt and pepper for taste

Directions:

1. Salt and pepper each breast. After pouring olive oil into slow cooker, place chicken into the slow cooker. Then, place onions on top, as well as all the herbs and garlic. Cover with tomatoes and vinegar.

2. Cook on high covered for 4 hours. Then, serve with pasta.

Deep Dish Cheese Pizza

Serves: 6

Nutritional Facts: Calories: 275 | Carbs: 4g | Protein: 18g | Fat: 21g

Ingredients:

Crust

- 1 ½ heads of cauliflower
- 3 eggs
- ¾ cup of cheese, shredded, Italian blend (63g)
- 1 ½ tsp. Italian seasoning
- ⅓ tsp. salt

Toppings

- ¾ cup of alfredo sauce, jarred (177ml)
- 2 ¼ cup of cheese, shredded, Italian blend (208g)
- ¾ tsp. rosemary, dried

Directions:

1. Chop up cauliflower heads and place them in a food processor. Pulse until diced and then add into a medium-sized mixing bowl. Add in the rest of the crust ingredients and mix them together.

2. Spray inside the slow cooker with non-stick spray and then press cauliflower mix into the bottom of the insert, making sure to bring the crust up a little on the sides.

3. Then, top with all the ingredients for the topping. Cover, leaving the lid a little gapped, and cook on high for 2-4 hours or until edges are lightly browned.

4. Turn off heat and let sit for half an hour. Then, cut and serve.

Pepper Jack Cauliflower

Serves: 6

Nutritional Facts: Calories: 272 | Carbs: 6.3g | Protein: 10.8g | Fat: 21.3g

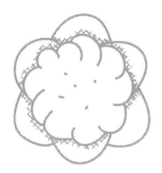

Ingredients:

♦ 1 head of cauliflower, cut into florets

♦ 4 oz. cream cheese (113g)

♦ ¼ cup of whipping cream (59ml)

♦ 2 tbsp. butter

♦ 1 tsp. salt

♦ ½ tsp. pepper

♦ 4 oz. pepper jack cheese, shredded (113g)

♦ 6 slices of bacon, cooked and crumbled

Directions:

1. Spray the inside of the slow cooker with non-stick cooking spray. Then, add all ingredients except cheese and bacon, combine well. Cook on low for 3 hours.

2. Then, add the cheese in and cook for another 30 minutes or until cauliflower is tender.

3. Serve garnished with bacon crumbles.

Slow Cooker Meatballs

Serves: 8

Nutritional Facts: Calories: 384 | Carbs: 10.7g | Protein: 32.7g | Fat: 21.7g

Ingredients:

Meatballs

- 1 lb. ground beef (454g)
- 1 lb. ground pork (454g)
- 1 large egg
- ¼ cup of mayonnaise (54g)
- ½ oz. pork rinds, crushed (14g)
- 2 tbsp. Parmesan cheese, grated
- 1 tsp. pepper
- 1 tsp. salt

Sauce

- 1 jar of chili sauce
- 1 jar of raspberry jam, sugar-free

Directions:

1. Turn slow cooker on high, cover and set aside. Preheat oven to 400 F (204 C). Then, grease a baking sheet with olive oil.

2. Combine all ingredients together until mixed well. Then, make meatballs (should make 42). Place them on a baking sheet and bake for about 15 minutes.

3. While they are baking, add all the sauce ingredients into the slow cooker and mix thoroughly.

4. Place baked meatballs in slow cooker and toss gently. Cover and cook on high for 2–3 hours. Serve.

Shrimp Tacos

Serves: 5

Nutritional Facts: Calories: 115 | Carbs: 5g | Protein: 14g | Fat: 2.5g

Ingredients:

♦ 1 lb. medium shrimp, peeled and deveined (454g)

♦ 1 tbsp. olive oil

♦ ½ cup of onion, chopped (89g)

♦ 1 can of fire-roasted diced tomatoes

♦ ½ cup of salsa, chunky (118ml)

♦ 1 bell pepper, chopped

♦ Salt and pepper for taste

♦ ½ tsp. cumin, ground

♦ ½ tsp. chili powder

♦ ¼ tsp. paprika

♦ 1 tsp. minced garlic

♦ 4 tbsp. cilantro, fresh, chopped

♦ Tortillas, paleo

Directions:

1. Place shrimp in the bottom of the slow cooker and then drizzle in olive oil and onion. Drain the fire-roasted tomatoes and pour into the slow cooker. Then, add in the rest of your ingredients and stir well.

2. Cover and cook on low for 2-3 hours or until shrimp is a nice pink color.

3. Remove from heat and serve in a tortilla with your choice of toppings.

Ginger Sesame Chicken

Serves: 8

Nutritional Facts: Calories: 220 | Carbs: 10g | Protein: 26g | Fat: 9g

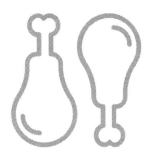

Ingredients:

♦ 1 ½ lbs. chicken breasts, boneless, skinless (680)
♦ ½ cup of tomato puree (158g)
♦ ⅓ cup of peach jam, unsweetened (104g)
♦ ⅓ cup of chicken broth (78ml)
♦ 2 tbsp. tamari sauce
♦ 1 ½ tbsp. honey
♦ 1 tsp. ginger, ground
♦ 2 cloves garlic, minced
♦ ¼ cup of onion, minced (43g)
♦ ½ tsp. red pepper flakes
♦ 2 tbsp. red bell pepper, chopped
♦ 1 ½ tbsp. scallions
♦ 2 tsp. sesame seeds

Directions:

1. Combine all ingredients (except chicken, bell peppers, scallions, and sesame seeds) into the slow cooker. Mix well and then toss in chicken. Stir until chicken is coated in sauce and sprinkle bell pepper over top.

2. Cover and cook on low for up to 6 hours. Then, serve over riced cauliflower and garnished with scallions and sesame seeds.

Sausage & Peppers

Serves: 6

Nutritional Facts: Calories: 365 | Carbs: 3g | Protein: 18g | Fat: 30g

Ingredients:

- ♦ 6 bratwurst
- ♦ 1 medium onion, chopped
- ♦ 2 bell peppers, chopped
- ♦ 2 cups of beef broth (473ml)
- ♦ ⅛ tsp. salt
- ♦ ½ tsp. pepper
- ♦ 2 tbsp. hot sauce

Directions:

1. Place all ingredients into the slow cooker and cook on low for 3 hours.
2. Remove from heat and serve with mashed cauliflower.

Pot Roast w/ Mushrooms

Serves: 6

Nutritional Facts: Calories: 634 | Carbs: 60g | Protein: 65g | Fat: 18g

Ingredients:

- 2 mushroom stock cubes
- 4 lb. Chuck roast, fat trimmed (1.8kg)
- 2 tbsp. steak rub
- 1 tsp. onion powder
- ¾ tsp. salt
- ½ tsp. pepper
- 3 tsp. olive oil
- 1 ½ lbs. mushrooms (680g)

Directions:

1. Trim the roast and cut it into sections. Then, dissolve mushroom cubes in water. Next, mix the steak rub, onion powder, salt, and pepper and then rub each side of the meat liberally.

2. In a large skillet, heat the oil and then sear each side of the pieces of meat. Transfer meat to the slow cooker. Use mushroom stock to deglaze the pan and then add that to the slow cooker, as well. Cover and cook on high for about 3 hours.

3. Then, add in mushrooms and let cook for another hour. Remove and plate meat and mushrooms, tenting with foil to keep warm.

4. Strain the juice into a saucepan and simmer to reduce. Then, serve with juice poured over the top.

Pork Loin Wrapped in Bacon

Serves: 4

Nutritional Facts: Calories: 247 | Carbs: .3g | Protein: 61g | Fat: 21.5g

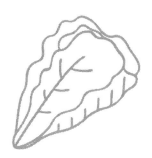

Ingredients:

- ♦ 2 lb. pork loin (907g)
- ♦ 4 strips of bacon
- ♦ 1 package of onion soup mix
- ♦ ¼ cup of water (59ml)

Directions:

1. Rub pork loin with onion soup mix. Pour the remaining soup mix into the slow cooker.

2. Wrap pork loin with the bacon and place it in the slow cooker. Then, pour the water in and cook on low for 7 hours.

3. Slice and serve.

Beef Short Ribs

Serves: 12

Nutritional Facts: Calories: 489 | Carbs: 3g | Protein: 16g | Fat: 42g

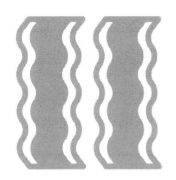

Ingredients:

- 4 lbs. beef short ribs (1.8kg)
- Salt and pepper for taste
- 3 tbsp. olive oil
- 1 cup of beef broth (237ml)
- 1 ½ cup of onion, chopped (256g)
- 3 cloves garlic, minced
- 2 tbsp. Worcestershire sauce
- 2 tbsp. tomato paste
- 1 ½ cup of red wine (355ml)

Directions:

1. Season one side of the short rib generously with salt and pepper. Then, heat the oil in a large skillet over medium-high heat and place short ribs in the skillet seasoned-side down. Then, season the other side and flip as needed. Repeat the process until all ribs have been browned.

2. Add beef broth into cooker and then place the ribs in. In the skillet used for the short ribs, add the rest of the ingredients and bring it to a boil. Cook for 5 minutes and then pour over ribs.

3. Cook on low for 8-10 hours with the lid on. Then, take out and serve.

LOW CARB RECIPES

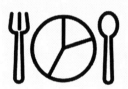

Mexican-Style Meatloaf

Serves: 8

Nutritional Facts: Calories: 222 | Carbs: 10g | Protein: 23g | Fat: 10g

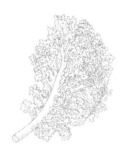

Ingredients:

♦ 6 tbsp. ketchup

♦ 2 tbsp. Worcestershire sauce

♦ 12 saltines, crushed

♦ 1 medium onion, chopped fine

♦ 6 cloves garlic, minced

♦ 1 tsp. paprika

♦ ½ tsp. salt

♦ ½ tsp. pepper

♦ ⅛ tsp. cayenne pepper

♦ 2 lb. of ground beef, lean (907g)

Directions:

1. Take two strips of aluminum foil and crisscross them in the slow cooker insert. Spray with non-stick cooking spray.

2. Combine all ingredients in a large mixing bowl and mix well. Then, shape into a round loaf and place in the slow cooker.

3. Cook on low for 4–5 hours or until no pink remains.

4. Remove, using foil as a lift, and place on platter. Cover top with ketchup, slice, and serve.

Coq au Vin

Serves: 4

Nutritional Facts: Calories: 299 | Carbs: 16g | Protein: 28g | Fat: 11g

Ingredients:

- 4 chicken breasts, boneless, skinless, halved
- 3 slices of bacon, chopped
- ½ lb. mushrooms, sliced (227g)
- 1 medium onion, chopped
- 4 cloves garlic, minced
- 1bay leaf
- ⅓ cup of flour, all-purpose (41g)
- ½ cup of red wine (118ml)
- ½ cup of chicken broth (118ml)
- ½ tsp. thyme, dried
- ¼ tsp. pepper

Directions:

1. Cook bacon until crisp in a large skillet over medium heat. Drain on paper towels. Then, add in chicken and brown on both sides. Place the chicken into the slow cooker.

2. Add the mushrooms, onions, and garlic to skillet and cook until tender. Cover chicken with mixture and add the bay leaf.

3. In a small mixing bowl, whisk together flour, wine, broth, thyme, and pepper until combined thoroughly. Then, pour this mixture over the chicken.

4. Cover and cook on low for 5-6 hours. Remove bay leaves and serve over rice or noodles.

Stuffed Cabbage Rolls

Serves: 6

Nutritional Facts: Calories: 204 | Carbs: 16g | Protein: 18g | Fat: 7g

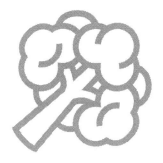

Ingredients:

- ♦ 12 cabbage leaves
- ♦ 1 cup of brown rice, cooked (178g)
- ♦ ¼ cup of onion, finely chopped (43g)
- ♦ 1 large egg
- ♦ ¼ cup of milk, fat-free (59ml)
- ♦ ½ tsp. salt
- ♦ ¼ tsp. pepper
- ♦ 1 lb. ground beef, lean (454g)

Sauce

- ♦ 1 can of tomato sauce
- ♦ 1 tbsp. brown sugar
- ♦ 1 tbsp. lemon juice, fresh
- ♦ 1 tsp. Worcestershire sauce

Directions:

1. Boil cabbage leaves in batches until just tender but still crisp. Drain and let cool for a few minutes. Then, trim the thick vein at the end and make a v-shaped cut. Cook beef in a skillet until just browned.

2. In a large mixing bowl, combine the cooked rice, onion, egg, milk, salt, and pepper. Combine thoroughly and then add the cooked beef. Then, place a few spoons full of that mixture in each leaf and fold cabbage over filling. Roll tightly.

3. Place rolls in slow cooker with the seam facing down. Mix sauce ingredients together in a medium mixing bowl and then pour over top.

4. Cook on low for 6-8 minutes. Then, remove from slow cooker and serve.

Pork and Butternut Squash Ragu

Serves: 10

Nutritional Facts: Calories: 195 | Carbs: 13g | Protein: 17g | Fat: 8g

Ingredients:

- 2 cans of stewed tomatoes
- 1 package of squash, frozen
- 1 large onion, diced large
- 1 medium red bell pepper, diced large
- 1 ½ tsp. red pepper flakes
- 2 lbs. pork ribs, boneless (907g)
- 1 tsp. salt
- ¼ tsp. garlic powder
- ¼ tsp. pepper

Directions:

1. Combine first 5 ingredients in the slow cooker. Then, season ribs with salt, garlic powder, and pepper and place in the slow cooker.

2. Cover and cook on low for 5-6 hours. Then, remove lid, stir the mixture to break up the pork, and then serve with pasta or rice topped with Parmesan cheese.

Apple-Dijon Pork Roast

Serves: 8

Nutritional Facts: Calories: 197 | Carbs: 11g | Protein: 23g | Fat: 7g

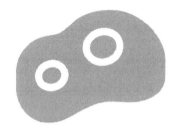

Ingredients:

♦ 1 pork loin, boneless

♦ 1 can of chicken broth

♦ 1 cup of apple juice, unsweetened (237ml)

♦ ½ cup of Dijon mustard (118ml)

♦ 6 tbsp. corn starch

♦ 6 tbsp. cold water

♦ Pepper and salt for taste

Directions:

1. Place pork loin in the slow cooker. Then, in a small mixing bowl, combine broth, apple juice, and mustard. Pour over pork and then cover. Cook on low for 4-5 hours or until tender. Remove roast and keep warm.

2. Strain the juice and get rid of fat. Place clarified juices into a small saucepan. Combine water and cornstarch until smooth and slowly stir mixture into juices. Bring to boil and stir continuously until thickened. Slice pork and serve with sauce drizzled over the top.

Swiss Steak

Serves: 6

Nutritional Facts: Calories: 171 | Carbs: 6g | Protein: 27g | Fat: 4g

Ingredients:

- ♦ 2 tbsp. flour, all-purpose
- ♦ ½ tsp. salt
- ♦ ¼ tsp. pepper
- ♦ 1 ½ lbs. beef round steak (680g)
- ♦ 1 medium onion, sliced
- ♦ 1 celery rib, sliced
- ♦ 2 cans of tomato sauce

Directions:

1. In a large freezer bag, combine flour, salt, and pepper. Shake until combined. Then, add the beef into the bag and repeat the shaking process.

2. Place onion on the bottom of the slow cooker and cover with the remaining ingredients. Make sure to shake the excess flour off of the beef.

3. Cover and cook on low for 6-8 hours and then serve.

Caribbean Curried Chicken

Serves: 8

Nutritional Facts: Calories: 249 | Carbs: 11g | Protein: 22g | Fat: 13g

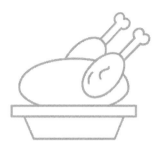

Ingredients:

- 1 tbsp. curry powder
- 1 tsp. garlic powder
- 1 tsp. pepper
- 8 chicken thighs, boneless, skinless
- 1 medium onion, sliced thin
- 1 ½ cups of mojo criollo marinade (355ml)
- 2 tbsp. canola oil
- 2 tbsp. flour, all-purpose

Directions:

1. Combine curry, garlic powder, and pepper, and then season chicken. Place chicken in the slow cooker and cover with onions. Then, pour the mojo criollo sauce along the sides of the cooker. Cook on low for 4-6 hours with the lid on. Remove the chicken and keep warm.

2. Pour juices through a fine-mesh strainer into a bowl. Then, heat a large saucepan with oil over medium heat and whisk flour into the oil until smooth. Slowly add the juice into the saucepan while whisking. Bring to a boil and let cook until thick. Next, add chicken and let simmer for another 5 minutes. Serve with rice and garnished with cilantro and/or scallions.

Lemon Garlic Chicken

Serves: 4

Nutritional Facts: Calories: 447 | Carbs: 7.9g | Protein: 63.4g | Fat: 16.8g

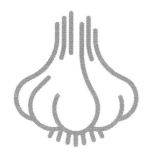

Ingredients:

- 1 tbsp. olive oil
- 4 chicken breasts, boneless, skinless
- ½ tsp. salt
- ¼ tsp. pepper
- 1 cup of chicken broth (237ml)
- ½ cup of lemon juice, fresh (118ml)
- 8 cloves garlic, smashed
- 2 tbsp. butter, unsalted
- 2 tbsp. flour, all-purpose
- Parsley, fresh, chopped

Directions:

1. In a large skillet over medium heat, add oil. Season chicken generously on all sides with salt and pepper and then sear in the skillet until lightly brown on both sides.
2. Place chicken in the slow cooker and add broth, lemon juice, and garlic. Cook on low for 3-4 hours.
3. In a medium mixing bowl, combine the butter and flour. Combine with fingers until smooth and then set to the side.
4. When chicken is done, place on a platter. Then, pour the liquid into a saucepan. Bring to a boil and then add the butter mixture, whisking until completely combined. Cook until sauce thickens and then pour over chicken. Serve garnished with parsley.

Ratatouille

Serves: 8 - 10

Nutritional Facts: Calories: 98 | Carbs: 11.4g | Protein: 2.2g | Fat: 5.8g

Ingredients:

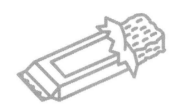

- 4 tbsp. olive oil
- 2 medium onions, diced
- 1 eggplant
- 2 zucchini
- 2 large bell peppers each red, green and yellow
- 1 lb. tomatoes (454g)
- 4 cloves garlic, smashed
- 2 tbsp. tomato paste
- ½ tsp. salt
- ¼ cup basil, fresh, chopped (21g)

Directions:

1. Heat 2 tbsp. of oil in a large skillet over medium heat. Add onions and cook until lightly browned. Cut up all the vegetables and place them in the slow cooker. Then, chop the garlic and add it, as well.

2. When onions are ready, add tomato paste and coat onions with it. Then, place this mixture into the slow cooker. Add the rest of the oil and salt. Stir the vegetables.

3. Cook on low for 5-6 hours with the lid on. If you need to get rid of some liquid, uncover and cook for half an hour more.

4. Stir in basil and serve drizzled with a little olive oil.

Pork Vindaloo

Serves: 6 - 8

Nutritional Facts: Calories: 624 | Carbs: 9.5g | Protein: 40.3g | Fat: 46.6g

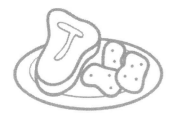

Ingredients:

- ♦ 1 piece of ginger, peeled
- ♦ 3 tbsp. canola oil
- ♦ ½ tsp. fenugreek seeds
- ♦ 3 medium onions, thinly sliced
- ♦ 4lbs. pork shoulder, cubed (1.8kg)
- ♦ 10 – 12 cloves garlic, minced
- ♦ 3 – 6 chilies, minced
- ♦ ½ tsp. turmeric, ground
- ♦ 2 tsp. Indian red chili, ground
- ♦ 1 ½ tsp. salt
- ♦ 2 tbsp. coriander seeds
- ♦ 1 tsp. cumin seeds
- ♦ ½ tsp. mustard seeds
- ♦ 4 cloves
- ♦ 3 cardamom pods
- ♦ 20 peppercorns
- ♦ 1 piece cassia
- ♦ 1 tsp. sugar
- ♦ 2 tbsp. tamarind paste
- ♦ 1 tbsp. white vinegar

Directions:

1. Turn slow cooker on to high and let heat for 15 minutes. Julienne 1" (2.5cm) of ginger. Reserve the rest of the ginger for garnish.

2. Heat the oil in a large skillet and then add in the fenugreek seeds. Add onions and cook until lightly browned. Then, add the onions into the slow cooker and mix in the pork, ginger, garlic, chili, turmeric, red chili, and salt. Cook on low for 3 ½ hours.

3. Grind coriander, cumin, mustard, cloves, cardamom, peppercorns, cassia, and sugar together in a spice grinder. Add spice blend and mix. Cook for another 30 minutes. Then, turn off slow cooker and stir in tamarind paste and vinegar. Serve garnished with julienned ginger.

Disclaimer

The opinions and ideas of the author contained in this publication are designed to educate the reader in an informative and helpful manner.

While we accept that the instructions will not suit every reader, it is only to be expected that the recipes might not gel with everyone. Use the book responsibly and at your own risk. This work with all its contents, does not guarantee correctness, completion, quality or correctness of the provided information. Always check with your medical practitioner should you be unsure whether to follow a low carb eating plan. Misinformation or misprints cannot be completely eliminated. Human error is real!

Cover: oliviaprodesign

Cover Photo: nadianb / shutterstock.com